HESI A2 Admission Exam Study Guide

Tanisha A. Wilson

ISBN: 1469954168
ISBN-13: 978-1469954165

DEDICATION

To Carlene Wilson, Mandy & John Broussard. My late mother and my maternal grandparents who always instilled in our family to get a good education. Also, to my entire family for their support. To my loving husband Francis and my two sons thanks for your love and belief in me.

CONTENTS

ACKNOWLEDGMENTS

Dr. Thomas my A&P professor
at Houston Community College. To all my teachers throughout my life.

1 ENGLISH-GRAMMAR USAGE

Cut the clutter. Cut the Cost. Ace the Test!

First the English portion of the HESI A2 test consists of three parts: correct usage of grammar, vocabulary, and reading comprehension.

HESI Hints: If it sounds incorrect it usually is.

They are eight parts of speech: nouns, pronouns, verbs, adjectives, adverbs, prepositions, conjunctions, and interjections.

Nouns: Is a word or group that signifies a person, place, or thing. They are four types of nouns include proper, common, abstract, and collective nouns.

Proper: Are always capitalize official names of person, places, or thing. **Example:** Texas

Common: Nouns that refer to general things. **Example:** girls

Abstract: Is the name a quality or general idea. **Example:** independence

Collective: Represents group of people, animal, or things. **Example:** homes

Pronouns: Is often defined as a word which can be used instead of a noun. Pronouns can be personal or possessive. Other types are indefinite, relative, interrogative, and demonstrative pronouns.

Personal pronouns: It often refers to a person. Like nouns, personal pronouns sometimes have singular and plural forms. **Example:** 1st person or the self (I, me, we), 2nd person or the person spoken to (you), 3rd person or the person spoken about (he, she, him, her, they, them).

Possessive pronouns: Shows ownership or possession. can stand by themselves without nouns. **Example:** mine, yours, his, hers.

Indefinite, relative, interrogative, and demonstrative pronouns: Interrogative pronouns (who, which, what) used for asking questions and relative pronouns (who, which, what, that) used in complex sentences which will be discussed in another place. Some grammar books also talk about demonstrative pronouns (this, that, these, those) and indefinite pronouns (some, all, both, each, etc.)

Adjectives: Is often defined as a word which describes or gives more information about a noun or pronoun. Adjectives describe nouns in terms of such qualities as size, color, number, and kind. **Example:** lazy, old, brown dog

Verbs: Is often defined as a word which shows action or state of being. The verb is the heart of a sentence- every sentence must have a verb. One of the most important things about verbs is their relationship to time. Verbs tell if something has already happened, if it will happen later, or if it is happening now.

Present, Past, and Future tense: For things happening now, we use the present tense of a verb; for something that has already happened, we use the past tense; and for something that will happen later, we use the future tense. **Example:** look, looked, will look

Adverbs: is usually defined as a word that gives more information about a verb, an adjective or another adverb. Adverbs describe verbs, adjectives and adverbs in terms of such qualities as time, frequency and manner. Most, but not all adverbs end in -ly as in But not all words that end in -ly are adverbs (ugly is an adjective, supply and reply can both be nouns or verbs). Many times an adjective can be made into an adverb by adding -ly as in nicely, quickly, completely, sincerely. Other examples: now, always, and twice.

Prepositions: is a word which shows relationships among other words in the sentence. The relationships include direction, place, time, cause, manner and amount. A preposition always goes with a noun or pronoun which is called the object of the preposition. The preposition is almost always before the noun or pronoun and that is why it is called a preposition. The preposition and the object of the preposition together are called a prepositional phrase.

Prepositions: The following chart shows the prepositions, objects of the preposition, and prepositional phrases of the sentences above.
Preposition
to/ by/ /at/ under
Object of the Preposition
the store/ bus/ three o'clock/ the table
Prepositional Phrase
to the store/ by bus/ at three o'clock/ under the table

Conjunctions: is a word that connects other words or groups of words. Conjunctions can be three types: coordinating, subordinating, and correlating.

Coordinating, subordinating, and correlating conjunctions: Coordinating conjunctions are conjunctions which connect two equal parts of a sentence. The most common ones are and, or, but, and so. Subordinating conjunctions connect two parts of a sentence that are not equal and will be discussed more in another class such as after, before, and it. Correlative conjunctions are pairs of conjunctions that work together such as either/or and both/and.

Interjections: Interjections are words used to express strong feeling or sudden emotion. They are included in a sentence - usually at the start - to express a sentiment such as surprise, disgust, joy, excitement or enthusiasm. **Example:** Hey! You get back here!

Important Grammar terms: Phrases can be part of a clause but a clause cannot be part of a phrase. A group of words that acts a part of a sentence.

Important Grammar terms: Clauses must contain a subject and a verb (simple predicate): a phrase need not. They are two types of clauses: independent and dependent

Important Grammar terms: If a clause can stand alone as a sentence, it is an independent clause, as in the following **Example:** The last stroke of twelve has ceased to vibrate.
They explain something else in the sentence. They depend upon that other part of the sentence because without it they do not make sense.
Example: When the last stroke of twelve has ceased to vibrate.

Important Grammar terms: When nouns are not subjects they are usually objects. When they are objects in relation to a verb they are who or what is receiving the action. They are on the other end of what happens when the subject joins the verb. Two types of objects are direct and indirect.

Important Grammar terms:
I'd give him a piece of my mind to feast upon
No doubt she told him her opinion.
In these two sentences "piece" and "opinion" are the direct objects. The "him" in each sentence is an indirect object. Indirect objects, like all objects, must be nouns or pronouns. Indirect objects answer the question to or for whom or what did the verb act upon.

Important Grammar terms: Predicate is the completer of a sentence. A simple predicate consists of only a verb, verb string, or compound verb:
The glacier melted.
The glacier has been melting.
The glacier melted, broke apart, and slipped into the sea.

Important Grammar terms: Predicate adjective follows a linking verb and tells us something about the subject:
Ramonita is beautiful.
His behavior has been outrageous.
That garbage on the street smells bad.

Important Grammar terms: Predicate nominative follows a linking verb and tells us what the subject is:
Dr. Couchworthy is acting president of the university.
She used to be the tallest girl on the team.

Important Grammar terms: Subject of a sentence is the person, place, thing, or idea that is doing or being something.

Important Grammar terms: a grammatical unit of one or more words, and typically expressing an independent statement, question, request, command, etc.,
Example: Summer is here. or Who is it? or Stop!

Common Grammar errors: Commas in a series: commas should be used to separate three or more elements in a series or list. **Example:** I went to the store to buy milk, bread, and eggs.

Common Grammar errors: Subject-verb agreement refers to ensuring that singular subjects have singular verbs, and plural subjects have plural verbs. This is called agreement in number, and it refers specifically to verbs in the present tense.
Example: (Subject-Verb—disagreement)
The dirty dishes sitting in the kitchen sink needs to be washed.
(Corrected)
The dirty dishes sitting in the kitchen sink need to be washed.

Common Grammar errors: Correct pronoun case requires different forms of personal pronouns for different jobs in sentences.

Common Grammar errors: The personal pronouns have 3 cases: subjective, objective, possessive

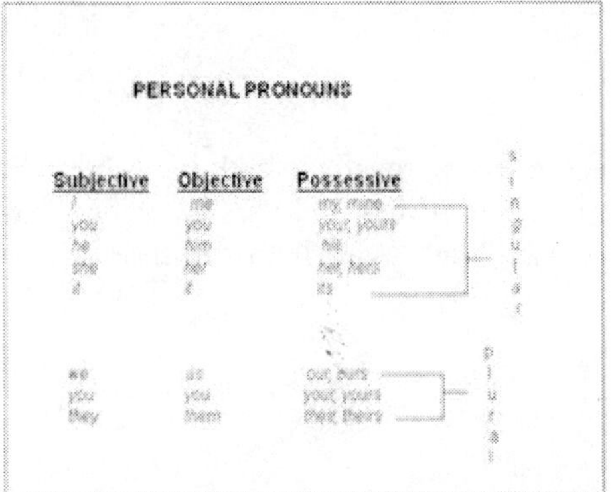

Common Grammar errors: In compound structures, where there are two pronouns or a noun and a pronoun, drop the other noun for a moment. Then you can see which case you want.

Not: Bob and me travel a good deal.

(Would you say, "me travel"?)
Not: He gave the flowers to Jane and I.
(Would you say, "he gave the flowers to I"

Common Grammar errors: In comparisons. Comparisons usually follow than or as:
He is taller than I (am tall).
This helps you as much as (it helps) me.
She is as noisy as I (am).

Common Grammar errors: In formal and semiformal writing:
Use the subjective form after a form of the verb to be.
Formal: It is I.
Informal: It is me.
Use whom in the objective case.
Formal: To whom am I talking?
Informal: Who am I talking to?

Common Grammar errors: (sometimes called a "fused sentence") has at least two parts, either one of which can stand by itself (in other words, two independent clauses), but the two parts have been smooshed together instead of being properly connected.

Common Grammar errors: It is important to realize that the length of a sentence really has nothing to do with whether a sentence is a run-on or not; being a run-on is a structural flaw that can plague even a very short sentence: The sun is high, put on some sunblock.

Common Grammar errors: An extremely long sentence, on the other hand, might be a "run-off-at-the-mouth" sentence, but it can be otherwise sound, structurally. When two independent clauses are connected by only a comma, they constitute a run-on sentence that is called a comma-splice. The example just above (about the sunscreen) is a comma-splice. When you use a comma to connect two independent clauses, it must be accompanied by a little conjunction (and, but, for, nor, yet, or, so). The sun is high, so put on some sunscreen.

Common Grammar errors: A compound sentence consists of two or more independent (main) clauses. Because the independent clauses in a compound sentence are grammatically equal structures, they are joined by one of the coordinating conjunctions (and, but, yet, or, nor, so) or by a set of correlatives (either-or, neither-nor, not only-but also, both-and).

Common Grammar errors: In general, when the independent clauses in a compound sentence are joined by a coordinating conjunction, they are separated by a comma. The comma precedes the coordinating conjunction. A common error is to place the comma after the conjunction:

WRONG: We picked them up early but, they still missed their plane.
RIGHT: We picked them up early, but they still missed their plane

Common Grammar errors: A sentence fragment occurs when an incomplete sentence is used instead of a complete sentence. Because there are common causes for sentence fragments, the following pointers may help in identifying and revising them: When using "ing" words, you must have a helping verb and a subject. An "ing" word is not a definite verb; therefore, it will not function by itself to form a complete sentence.
Fragment
A cure for the disease being researched
Sentence
A cure for the disease was being researched.

Common Grammar errors: An infinitive form of a verb will not make a complete sentence. Like "ing" words, an infinitive is not a definite verb either. An infinitive is the combination of to and the base form of a verb: to see, to be, to do. Infinitives are used in sentences, but they require a definite verb to function as the action in the sentence.
Fragment

The center to plan a mission statement.
Sentence
The center plans to develop a mission statement.

Common Grammar errors: Subordinators are words that cause one part of a sentence to be dependent on another part of the sentence. They can be a cause of sentence fragments if they subordinate a clause that does not have a main clause for the subordinate clause to be dependent upon.
Fragment
If the criteria are not met.
Sentence
If the critieria are not met, the FDA will not approve the medicine.

Common Grammar errors: An explanatory phrase or group of explanatory words does not make a complete sentence on its own.
Fragment
The teenagers like to watch sports. Such as hockey, when they are on television.
Sentence
The teenagers like to watch sports, such as hockey, when they are on television.

2 ENGLISH-READING COMPREHENSION

HESI tip: This part consist of 4 to 5 short stories

Reading Comprehension: A paragraph is a group of sentences related to a particular topic, or central theme. Every paragraph has a key concept or main idea. The main idea is the most important piece of information the author wants you to know about the concept of that paragraph. When authors write they have an idea in mind that they are trying to get across. This is especially true as authors compose paragraphs. An author organizes each paragraph's main idea and supporting details in support of the topic or central theme, and each paragraph supports the paragraph preceding it. A writer will state his/her main idea explicitly somewhere in the paragraph. That main idea may be stated at the beginning of the paragraph, in the middle, or at the end. The sentence in which the main idea is stated is the topic sentence of that paragraph.

Reading Comprehension: Supporting details are the facts and ideas that explain or prove the topic sentence or main idea. These sentences have information that helps explain and prove the author's point. For example, a paragraph about how animals hide might have supporting details about camouflage. Strong paragraphs have clear and organized details that relate to the main idea.

Reading Comprehension: Using context cues to figure out a word's meaning is like being a detective. The reader comes across a mystery—an unknown word—and has to use clues to solve it. The clues might be words before the mystery word, after it or even in the following sentence. It requires careful thinking, rereading and fact checking.
Here's one theory one how to use context clues:
"To Use Context Clues"
1. Look for clues, or hints, around a word you don't know.
2. Use the clues to guess a meaning for the word.

Reading Comprehension:
Definition-the word is defined directly and clearly in the sentence in which it appears.
Example: The arbitrator, the neutral person chosen to settle the dispute, arrived at her decision.
Antonym (or contrast)-often signaled by the words whereas, unlike, or as opposed to.
Example: Unlike Jamaal's room, which was immaculate, Jeffrey's room was very messy.

Reading Comprehension: Synonym (or restatement)-other words are used in the sentence with similar meanings.
Example: The slender woman was so thin her clothes were too big on her.
Inference-word meanings are not directly described, but need to be inferred from the context.
Example: Walt's pugnacious behavior made his opponent back down.

Reading Comprehension:
Explanation : The unknown word is explained within the sentence or in a sentence immediately preceding.
Example: The patient is so somnolent that she requires medication to help her stay awake for more than a short time
Examples: Specific examples are used to define the term.
Example: Celestial bodies, such as the sun, moon, and stars, are governed by predictable laws."

Reading Comprehension: Every written piece of information is created by an author who has a specific reason for writing. This reason for writing is known as the author's purpose. Effective readers read to understand the author's purpose. Understanding purpose is closely related to the ability to identify the tone of a passage. Tone is the emotion or mood of the author's written voice. Purpose and tone are established with word choice.

Reading Comprehension: From a very traditional standpoint you could say that a fact is something that is objectively true and that does not alter depending on the perspective or perception of the person observing it. For example you could say today is Friday, the leaf is green or 2 plus 2 equals four. An opinion is where someone puts his or her perspective into the picture. Thank goodness it is Friday, I like Friday because it is nearly the weekend. I like a particular TV show, or I think it is hot outside.

Reading Comprehension: Inference is the act or process of deriving a conclusion based solely on what one already knows. Making an inference is also known as reading between the lines. The reader must put together the information the author provides and the information that the reader already knows to come up with the answer. Deductive reasoning, finding the effect with the cause and the rule. Abductive reasoning, finding the cause with the rule and the effect. Inductive reasoning, finding the rule with the cause and the effect.

Reading Comprehension:
Here are some guidelines for summarizing a passage.
Read the given passage to find:
1. What the passage is about.
2. What its tone is.
3. What type of writing it is.

Notes:

Vocabulary and General Knowledge:
A suffix is simply an ending that's added to a base word to form a new word.

Let's look at some examples:
Base word Suffix New Word
interest -   ing   interesting
noise   -y   noisy
breath   -less   breathless
popular   -ity   popularity
drop   -let   droplet
A key thing to know about a suffix is whether it starts with a consonant or a vowel.

Vocabulary and General Knowledge:
Analogy is just a term that means "word relationships".
Analogies are sometimes formatted as follows:
[word 1] : [word 2] : : [word 3] : [word 4]
In this analogy format,: reads "is to" and : : reads "as"
This means that
water: liquid : : ice : solid is read as
Water is to liquid as ice is to solid.

HESI hint: the vocabulary comes in to two forms it will asked for the word directly or the meaning in a sentence.
Example: What does urinate mean?
Example: The patient felt an acute feeling of nausea today. What does acute means in this sentence.

Vocabulary and General Knowledge:
ABRUPT= sudden change with warning
ABSTAIN= to refrain from something by one's choice
ACCESS= a means to obtain entry or a means of approach
ACCOUNTABLE= responsible
ADHERE= to hold fast or stick together
ADVERSE= undesired, possibly harmful
AFFECT= appearance of observable emotions
ANNUAL= happening once a year
APPLY= to place, put on, or spread something
AUDIBLE= able to be heard
BILATERAL= present on two sides
CAST= hard protective device applied to protect a broken bone while it heals
CEASE= come to an end or bring to an end
COMPENSATORY= offsetting or making up for something
COMPLICATION= an undesired problem that is the result of some other event
COMPLY= do as directed
CONCAVE= rounded inward like a bowl
CONCISE= brief, to the point
CONSISTENCY= degree of viscosity
CONSTRICT= to draw together or become smaller
CONTINGENT= dependent on something to happen
CONTOUR= shape or outline of shape
CONTRACT= to draw together or reduce in size

CONTRAINDICATION= a reason why something is not advisable or why it should not be done
DEFECATE= expel feces
DEFICIT= a deficiency or lack of something
DEPRESS= press downward
DEPTH= downward measurement from the surface
DETERIORATING= worsening
DEVICE= tool or piece of equipment
DIAMETER= The distance across the center of an object
DILUTE= to make a liquid less concentrated
DISCRETE= distinct, separate
DISTENDED= enlarged or expanded from pressure
ELEVATE= to place in a higher position
ENDOGENOUS= produced within the body
EXACERBATE= to make worse
EXCESS= more than what is needed or usual
EXOGENOUS= produced outside the body
EXPAND= to increase in size or amount
EXPOSURE= contact, making secret known
EXTERNAL= located outside the body
FATAL= resulting in death
FATIGUE= extreme tiredness
FLACCID= limp, lacking tone
FLUSHED= reddened or ruddy appearance
GAPING= wide open
GENDER= sex of an individual
HYDRATION= maintenance of body fluid balance
HYGIENE= measures contributing to cleanliness and good health
IMPAIRED= diminished or lacking some usual quality or level
IMPENDING= likely to occur soon
INCIDENCE= occurrence
INFLAMED= reddened, swollen, warm and often tender
INGEST= to swallow for digestion
INITIATE= to begin or put into practice
INSIDIOUS= so as to not become apparent for a long time
INTACT= in place, unharmed
INTERNAL= located within the body or mind
INVASIVE= inserting or entering into the body part
LABILE= changing rapidly and often
LATENT= present, but not active or visible
LETHARGIC= difficult to arouse
MANIFESTATION= an indication or sign of a condition
NUTRIENT= substance or ingredient that provides nutrition
OCCLUDED= closed or obstructed
OMINOUS= significantly important or dangerous
ONGOING= continuous
ORAL= given through or affecting the mouth
OVERT= obvious or easily observed
PARAMETER= a characteristic or constant factor
PAROXYSMAL= beginning suddenly or abruptly
PATENT= conveys ownership of idea or invention
POTENT= giving a strong effect
POTENTIAL= capable of occurring or likely to occur
PRECAUTION= preventive measure

PRECIPITOUS= rapid, uncontrolled
PREDISPOSE= to make more susceptible or likely to occur
PREEXISTING= already exists
PRIMARY= first or most significant
PRIORITY= of great importance
PROGNOSIS= the anticipated or expected course of outcome
RATIONALE= the underlying reason
RECUR= to occur again
RESTRICT= to limit
RETAIN= to hold or keep
SITE= location or physical space
STATUS= condition or risk
STRICT= stringent, exact, complete
SUPPLEMENT= to take in addition to or to complete
SUPPRESS= to stop or subdue
SYMMETRIC= being equal or the same size shape and position
SYMPTOM= an indication of a problem
UNTOWARD=adverse or negative
URINATE= excrete or expel urine
VERBAL= spoken, using words
VITAL= essential to life
VOID= excrete, expel urine
VOLUME= amount of space occupied by a fluid

Notes:

Good Luck on your test!

4 MATH-ADDITION, SUBTRACTION, MULTIPLICATION, & DIVISION

First the Math portion of the HESI A2 test consists of 50 questions. These questions consist of basic mathematics which includes addition, subtraction, multiplication, division, fractions, decimals, percents, ratio and proportion, and other general math facts.

Let's get started!

First we will start with basic addition:
Line up the numbers to their place value.
Place value: where each number occupies a space. ones, tens, hundreds and so on. Add numbers from right to left:
1,200 + 800= add ones: 0 + 0= 0
add tens: 0 + 0=0
add hundreds: 2 + 8=10 carry over 1
add thousands: 1 + 1= 2
Answer= 2,000

Let's practice some addition problems:
1. 2,649 + 500=
2. 802 + 219=
3. 100 + 30 + 5=
4. 10,200 + 1,005=
5. 1,800 + 299=
Answer Key:
1. 3,149
2. 1,021
3. 135
4. 11,205
5. 2,009

First we will start with basic subtraction:

Line up the numbers to their place value.
Place value: where each number occupies a space. ones, tens, hundreds and so on
Subtract numbers from right to left:
977 - 890=
subtract ones: 7 - 0 = 7
subtract tens: 7 - 9= must borrow 1 from the number 9 making it 17 - 9=8
subtract hundreds: 8 - 8=0
Answer= 87

Let's practice some subtraction problems:
1. 100 - 60=
2. 12,356 - 2,345=
3. 2,001 - 500=
4. 150,000 - 25,660=
5. 14,000 - 450=

Answer Key:
1. 40
2. 10,011
3. 1,501
4. 124,340
5. 13,550

Next basic multiplication: The operation by which the product of two quantities is calculated. Line up numbers and multiply by place value. Don't forget to add placeholders when multiplying more two numbers. Placeholders=holds the ones place on multiplication and keeps problem align. Multiply from right to left.
200 x 12=
200
x12
400-ones
+2000-hundreds with placeholder 0
Answer: 2400

Let's practice some multiplication problems:
1. 10,230 x 230=
2. 1,340 x 12=
3. 500 x 23=
4. 23,340 x 4 =
5. 200,340 x 456=
Answer Key:
1. 2,352,900
2. 16,080
3. 11,500
4. 93,360
5. 91,355,040

Next basic division: All division problems involve four numbers: the dividend, the divisor, the quotient and the remainder. The dividend is the number that is being divided. The divisor is the number by which the dividend is divided. The quotient is the number of times that the divisor wholly goes in to the dividend. The remainder is the number that is left over from the divisor. The remainder must be either zero or a number less than the divisor.
Divide 200÷4= 4 ÷ 200=use a combo of multi. and add.
4 x 5=20
20 - 20=0
Answer=50 to check just multiply 50x4=200

Let's practice some division problems:
1. 10,000 ÷ 100=
2. 1,200 ÷ 4=
3. 250 ÷ 12=
4. 350,000 ÷ 1,000=
5. 22,250 ÷ 50=
Answer Key:
1. 100
2. 300
3. 20.833
4. 350
5. 445

5 MATH-FRACTIONS

Since you are entering into the healthcare field fractions are very important. Math fractions are numbers that are expressed as the ratio of two numbers. We will discuss terms, improper/mixed fractions, reducing, and least common denominator. Also how to add, subtract, multiply, and division of fractions.

Terms:
A fraction is a number that represents part of a whole.
A fraction consists of a numerator and a denominator, the numerator representing a number of equal parts and the denominator telling how many of those parts make up a whole.
For example, 2/7 is a fraction and 2 is the numerator and 7 is the denominator. (Source: From Wikipedia).

Types of Fractions: There are three types of fractions
Proper Fractions: The numerator is less than the denominator
Examples: 1/3, 3/4, 2/7
Improper Fractions: The numerator is greater than (or equal to) the denominator.
Examples: 4/3, 11/4, 7/7
Mixed Fractions: A whole number and proper fraction together.
Examples: 1 1/3, 2 1/4, 16 2/5

Addition of fractions is one of the important mathematical operations of fractions. To add together two fractions, first we need to find equivalent fractions that share a common denominator, then the sum is given by adding the numerators.

There are two kinds of addition of fractions:
Add fractions with same denominators
Add fractions with different denominators

Add fractions with same denominators:
Make sure the bottom numbers (the denominators) are the same. Add the top numbers (the numerators). Put the answer over the same denominator. The denominators will remain the denominator of the built up fraction. Simplify or reduce the fraction (if needed)
Example:
2/5 + 1/5=
Solution
Here the problem is to add 2/5 and 1/5
The denominators of the given fractions are same.
So we just add the numerator and the denominator remains unchanged.
2/5 + 1/5 = 2+1/5= 3/5

Adding fractions with different denominators:
Find the Least Common Denominator (LCD) of the fractions. Rename the fractions to have the LCD. Add the numerators of the fractions. Simplify the Fraction (if needed)
Example: Add the fraction 1/3 and 5/8=
LCD for 3 and 8 is 24.
First fraction: 1/3 x 8/8=8/24
Second fraction: 5/8 x 3/3=15/24
Add fractions together: 8/24 + 15/24
Answer= 23/24

Subtraction of fractions is one of the important mathematical operations of fractions. To subtract together two fractions, first we need to find equivalent fractions that share a common denominator, then the sum is given by subtracting the numerators.

There are two kinds of subtraction of fractions:
Subtract fractions with same denominators
Subtract fractions with different denominators

Subtraction of Fractions with Like denominators:
Bottom denominators should be same. Subtract the numerator place answer over same denominator in step above. Now, simplify the fraction if needed.
Example: 7/8 - 1/8= 6/8 simplify to 3/4

Subtract fractions with different denominators:
Build each fraction so that both denominators are equal. Remember, when subtracting fractions, the denominators must be equal. So we must complete this step first. Most of the time you will be required to work the problem using what's called the Least Common Denominator (LCD). In either case you will build each fraction into an equivalent fraction. Re-write each equivalent fraction using this new denominator. Now you can subtract the numerators, and keep the denominator of the equivalent fractions. When you borrow for subtraction, remember to reduce the whole number by one and add the denominator to the numerator giving you a new numerator quantity. Therefore 4 1/4 becomes 3 5/4. Always reduce your answer to its lower terms. Remember to move the whole number then reduce the fraction (4 4/8 = 4 1/2) it sometimes helps to place the reducing number between equal lines. Now, simplify the fraction if needed.
Example: 1/2 - 1/5= LCD is 10
5/10 - 2/10= 3/10

Let's practice some add./sub. fraction problems:
1. 1/4 + 3/4=
2. 1/3 + 3/8=
3. 1 1/2 + 2 5/9=
4. 3/4 - 1/4=
5. 5/6 - 1/6
6. 3 1/3 - 2 4/5=
Answer Key:
1. 4/4 or 1
2. 17/24
3. 4 1/18
4. 2/4=1/2
5. 4/6=2/3
6. 8/15

Multiplying fractions:
Always write the problem as given. Convert any mixed numbers into improper fractions. Multiply the numerators. Multiply the denominators. Always reduce your answer to its lower terms. Remember to move the whole number then reduce the fraction (3 4/8 = 3 1/2) it sometimes helps to place the reducing number between equal lines. Always write the problem as given. Convert any mixed numbers into improper fractions. Multiply the numerators. Multiply the denominators. Always reduce your answer to its lower terms. Remember to move the whole number then reduce the fraction (3 4/8 = 3 1/2) it sometimes helps to place the reducing number between equal lines.
Example: 2 2/9 x 3/12=
20/9 x 3/12= 60/81=30/27=10/9= 1 1/9

Let's practice multiplying fraction problems:
1. 2/5 x 3/8=
2. 1/4 x 5/6=
3. 4 1/2 x 1/6=
4. 7/8 x 1/4=
5. 2 5/6 x 3 1/3=

Answer Key:
1. 3/20
2. 5/24
3. 3/4
4. 7/32
5. 9 4/9

Dividing fractions:
Invert the denominator fraction and multiply the fractions. Multiply the numerators of the fractions. Multiply the denominators of the fractions. Place the product of the numerators over the product of the denominators. Simplify the Fraction
Example: Divide 2/9 and 3/12
Invert the denominator fraction and multiply (2/9 ÷ 3/12 = 2/9 x 12/3)
Multiply the numerators (2 x 12=24)
Multiply the denominators (9 x 3=27)
Place the product of the numerators over the product of the denominators (24/27)
Simplify the Fraction (24/27 = 8/9)

Multiplying two mixed numbers: Convert each mixed number to an improper fraction. Multiply the two numerators together. Multiply the two denominators together. Convert the result back to a mixed number if it is an improper fraction. Simplify the mixed number.
Dividing Fractions with Mixed Numbers:
Example: 6 2/8 ÷ 3 5/9 =
Convert each mixed number to an improper fraction. 50/8 ÷ 32/9
Invert the improper fraction that is the divisor and multiply. 50/8 x 9/32
Multiply the two numerators together. 50 x 9 = 450
Multiply the two denominators together. 8 x 32 = 256
Convert the result back to a mixed number. 450/256 = 1 194/256
Simplify the mixed number. 1 97/128

Let's practice dividing fraction problems:
1. 1/3 ÷ 3/4=
2. 5/7 ÷ 10/15=
3. 1 5/8 ÷ 9/27=
4. 4/5 ÷ 2/3=
5. 3 3/10 ÷ 1 1/10=
Answer Key:
1. 4/9
2. 1 1/14
3. 4 7/8
4. 1 1/5
5. 3

6-MATH-DECIMALS, PERCENTS, & CONVERSION

Decimals: A decimal is any number in our base-ten number system. Specifically, we will be using numbers that have one or more digits to the right of the decimal point. The decimal point is used to separate the ones place from the tenths place in decimals. As we move to the right of the decimal point, each number place is divided by 10.

Example: 1 1/4 = 1.25 divide 1/4 to show the fractional part as a decimal and leave the whole number 1 as is. As with whole numbers, a digit in a decimal number has a value which depends on the place of the digit. The places to the left of the decimal point are ones, tens, hundreds, and so on, just as with whole numbers.

This table shows the decimal place value for various positions: Note that adding extra zeros to the right of the last decimal digit does not change the value of the decimal number.

Place (underlined)

Name of Position

1 = Ones (units) position

1.2 = Tenths

1.23 = Hundredths

1.234 = Thousandths

1.2345 = Ten thousandths

1.23456 = Hundred Thousandths

1.234567 = Millionths

Adding Decimals: To add decimals, line up the decimal points and then follow the rules for adding or subtracting whole numbers, placing the decimal point in the same column as above. When one number has more decimal places than another, use 0's to give them the same number of decimal places.

Example: 76.75 + 51.40=

1) Line up the decimal points:

76.75 + 51.40=

2) Then add.

 76.75 + 51.40= 128.15

Subtracting Decimals: To subtract decimals, line up the decimal points and then follow the rules for adding or subtracting whole numbers, placing the decimal point in the same column as above. When one number has more decimal places than another, use 0's to give them the same number of decimal places.

Example: 18.25 - 6.009=

1) Line up the decimal points.

18.25 - 6.009=

2) Add extra 0's, using the fact that 18.25 = 18.250

18.250 - 6.009=

3) Subtract.

18.250 - 6.009=12.241

Let's practice subtracting and adding decimals problems:

1. 1.4 + 1.5=

2. 100.990 + 25.65=

3. 25000.6987 + 55509.578=

4. 2.1 - 0.9=

5. 1000.234 - 650.75=

6. 50000.4569 - 3069.065=

Answer Key:
1. 2.9
2. 126.64
3. 80510.2767
4. 1.2
5. 349.484
6. 46931.3919

Multiplying decimals: Multiply the numbers just as if they were whole numbers. Line up the numbers on the right - do not align the decimal points. Starting on the right, multiply each digit in the top number by each digit in the bottom number, just as with whole numbers. Add the products. Place the decimal point in the answer by starting at the right and moving a number of places equal to the sum of the decimal places in both numbers multiplied.
Example:
4.77 x 2.8=
3816 + 954=13.356 moved three decimal places

Dividing decimals: If the divisor is not a whole number, move decimal point to right to make it a whole number and move decimal point in dividend the same number of places. Divide as usual. Keep dividing until the answer terminates or repeats. Put decimal point directly above decimal point in the dividend. Place the divisor before the division bracket and place the dividend (0.4131) under it.
0.170 ÷ .4131=
Multiply both the divisor and dividend by 100 so that the divisor is not a decimal but a whole number. In other words move the decimal point two places to the right in both the divisor and dividend.
17 ÷ 41.31=
Proceed with the division as you normally would except put the decimal point in the answer or quotient exactly above where it occurs in the dividend.
17 ÷ 41.31=2.43

Let's practice multiplying and dividing decimals problems:
1. 0.010 x 5.50=
2. 90.64 x 6=
3.780.26 x .002=
4. 49 ÷ 0.7=
5. 0.81 ÷ 0.9=
6. 50.05 ÷ .005=
Answer Key:
1. 0.055
2. 543.84
3. 1.56052
4. 70
5. 0.9
6. 10010

Percentages: a percentage is a way of expressing a number as a fraction of 100 or "per hundred"
Example: 50% is 50/100 or .50.
Percent formula: is used to find percentages and fairly easy to to use. is/of = %/100
An important thing to remember: Cross multiply
Example: What is 9 out of 10 as a percent?
(rework with percent formula) 9/10 = %/100=
Cross multiply: 9 x 100= 900
Divide with remaining number.
900 ÷ 10= 90%

Let's practice percentage problems:
1. 25 % of 200 is_____ .
2. What number is 2% of 50?
3. ___% of 45 is 9
4. What is 20 out of 40 as a percent?
5. 24% of___ is 36.
Answer Key:
1. 50
2. 1
3. 20
4. 50
5. 150

Converting decimals, fractions, and percentages.
Percent to Decimal: move the decimal point to places to right.
Example: 75% = .75
Percent to Fraction: Convert the percent to a decimal, and then to a fraction.
Example: 60%= .60= 60/100

Converting decimals, fractions, and percentages.
Decimal to Fraction: First, convert the decimal to fraction using tenths, hundredths, thousandths, etc. depending on the number of decimal places.
Example: 1.75 = 1 75/100. Next, simplify the fraction part to the lowest common term.
Example: 75/100 = 3/4
Decimal to Percentage: just move the decimal point two places to the right.
Example: .65= 65%

Converting decimals, fractions, and percentages.
Fraction to Decimal: Divide the numerator by the denominator. The numerator is the number above a fraction line. The denominator is the number below the fraction line. In the fraction 2/100, two is the numerator and 100 is the denominator. Identify recurring numbers. Recurring numbers occur when the answer to the equation is infinite. Example: 1/3 is 0.3333333 and so on.
Fraction to Percent: Find a number you can multiply the bottom of the fraction by to get 100. Multiply both top and bottom of the fraction by that number. Then write down just the top number with the "%" sign. Example: 3/4 as a percent. We can multiply 4 by 25 to become 100. Multiply top and bottom by 25= 3/4 = 75/100. Write down 75 with the percent sign= 75%

Let's practice some problems.
1. Write 86% as a decimal.
2. Write 0.5 as a percentage.
3. Write 2/10 as a percentage.
4. Write 50% as a fraction.
5. Write 614/100,000 as a decimal.
Answer Key:
1. 0.86
2. 50%
3. 20%
4. 1/2
5. .00614

Chart of decimals, fraction, and percentages equivalent.
Fraction Decimal Percent
1/2 0.5 50%
1/3 0.333... 33.333...%
2/3 0.666... 66.666...%
1/4 0.25 25%

3/4 0.75 75%
1/5 0.2 20%
2/5 0.4 40%
3/5 0.6 60%
4/5 0.8 80%

Chart of decimals, fraction, and percentages equivalent.
Fraction Decimal Percent
1/6 0.1666... 16.666...%
5/6 0.8333... 83.333...%
1/8 0.125 12.5%
3/8 0.375 37.5%
5/8 0.625 62.5%
7/8 0.875 87.5%

Chart of decimals, fraction, and percentages equivalent.
Fraction Decimal Percent
1/9 0.111... 11.111...%
2/9 0.222... 22.222...%
4/9 0.444... 44.444...%
5/9 0.555... 55.555...%
7/9 0.777... 77.777...%
8/9 0.888... 88.888...%

Chart of decimals, fraction, and percentages equivalent.
Fraction Decimal Percent
1/10 0.1 10%
1/12 0.08333 8.333...%
1/16 0.0625 6.25%
1/32 0.03125 3.125%

Notes:

7 MATH-RATIO &PROPORTION/WORD PROBLEMS

Ratio and Proportions: A ratio is a comparison of two numbers. A proportion is an equation with a ratio on each side. It is a statement that two ratios are equal. Example: Write the ratio of 8 and 12. We can write this as 8:12 or as a fraction 8/12, and we say the ratio is eight to twelve. 3/4 = 6/8 is an example of a proportion.

HESI Hint: Practice ratio and proportions very often.

Let's practice ratio and proportion problems:
1. 10/91 show as a ratio.
2. 0.025 show as a ratio.
3. 2 : x = 3 : 9
4. 4 : 9 = 8 : x
5. 2 : 9 = x : 72
6. 360 : 60 = 6 : x
Answer Key:
1. 10:91 or 10 to 91
2. 25/1000=1/40=1:40 or 1 to 40
3. x= 6
4. x= 18
5. x= 16
6. x= 1

The HESI Math test has various word problems using the math we have reviewed already especially ratio and proportion. Here are examples of some word problems to be familiar with.

Solve the following word problem: Two cars leave two different cities located 957 miles apart at the same time. Car A is traveling at 70 miles per hr and Car B is traveling at 60 miles per hr. How many hours will it take for the two cars to meet? This is distance problem and you need to use distance formula. distance= rate x time or d=rt. You have the rate and must multiply to find the time which is unknown.
70(t) + 60(t)= 957
130(t) = 957 divide both sides by 130
t= 7.36 hours make sure you pay attention to look for 7.36 hours not 7.36 which is not correct

Word problems: Solve the following word problem: Michael and Carlen are brothers. Michael is 6 years older than Carlen. Michael was born in 1999. In what year was Carlen born. This problem is a simple addition problem. x= 1999
the year Michael was born
x +6= the year Carlen was born , he is six years younger.
1999 + 6= 2005 make sure you put the year and not his age.

Word Problems: Solve the following word problem: Assume that state tax is 8.25%. Francis purchases a new dining table that cost $450. What is the total cost with tax included? This problem is calculating total cost of a item. You must convert the percent to decimal 8.25% to 0.0825, if not you will get the wrong answer. $450 + ($450)8.25%= total cost. $450 + $37.125= $487.13. Make sure you have the dollar sign in the answer. Again pay attention

Word Problems: Solve the following word problem: Cedra uses a comic book store to sell comic books. Over the last week, she has sold books for $8, $26, $50, $70, and $20. What is the average price of the comic books sold by Cedra? This problem is mean (average) problem. $8, $26, $50, $70, and $20 ÷ 5= $34.80 Make sure you have the dollar sign in the answer.

Word Problems: Solve the following word problem: What is the simple interest on $40,000 invested at 15% annual rate over 4 years? This problem uses the formula for calculating simple interest. interest= principal x rate x time. $40,000 x .15 x 4= $24,000

Word Problems: Solve the following word problem: Jarvis's parents gave him 650 shares of stock in X company. Jarvis will receive $25.75 per share in dividend payout each year. How much will Jarvis earn in dividends over a two year period? This is multiplication problem. First you must get the dividends for the first year. Secondly, get the dividends for two years. $25.75 x 650= $16,737.50 $16,737.50 x 2= $33475

Word Problems: Solve the following word problem: George buys a tablet PC on sale. The original price of the tablet PC is $250. He paid $150. What is the discount on the tablet PC? This is a percent change problem. This formula will be used: amount of change ÷ original amount. You must find the difference between the amounts given in order to complete the problem. $250-$150=$100. 100/250= 0.40 or 40%

Word Problems: Solve the following word problem: Cindy's is preparing for a party. If her recipe calls for 5 pounds of ground beef and 10 pounds of lasagna noodles to serve 20, how many pounds will she need to feed 200 people? This is ratio and proportion problem. Set up proportions. Then, cross multiply. 5/20= x/200. 20x=1000. x=50 pounds. Note: these types of problems may have not always whole number.

Notes:

8 MEASUREMENTS US-METRIC & GENERAL FACTS

Metric Conversion: In healthcare you will have to get use to using the metric system instead of the US version. Here are common measurements used throughout the healthcare system.

Length
10 millimeters (mm) = 1 centimeter (cm)
10 centimeters = 1 decimeter (dm) = 100 millimeters
10 decimeters = 1 meter (m) = 1,000 millimeters
10 meters = 1 dekameter (dam)
10 dekameters = 1 hectometer (hm) = 100 meters
10 hectometers = 1 kilometer (km) = 1,000 meters

Area
100 square millimeters (mm2) = 1 sq centimeter (cm2)
10,000 square centimeters = 1 sq meter (m2)=1,000,000 sq millimeters
100 square meters =1 are (a)
100 acres =1 hectare (ha)=10,000 sq meters
100 hectares =1 sq. kilometer (km2)=1,000,000 sq meters

Volume
10 milliliters (ml) = 1 centiliter (cl)
10 centiliters = 1 deciliter (dl) = 100 milliliters
10 deciliters = 1 liter (l) = 1,000 milliliters
10 liters = 1 dekaliter (dal)
10 dekaliters = 1 hectoliter (hl) = 100 liters
10 hectoliters = 1 kiloliter (kl) = 1,000 liters

Weight
10 milligrams (mg) =1 centigram (cg)
10 centigrams =1 decigram (dg)= 100 milligrams
10 decigrams =1 gram (g)= 1,000 milligrams
10 grams =1 dekagram (dag)
10 dekagrams =1 hectogram (hg)= 100 grams
10 hectograms =1 kilogram (kg)= 1,000 grams
1,000 kilograms =1 metric ton (t)

US-Metric Conversion: you will have word problems with conversions and will need to know this information.

Length
mile-mi=5280 feet, 1760 yards, 320 rods=1.609 kilometers
rod-rd=5.50 yards, 16.5 feet=5.029 meters
yard-yd=3 feet, 36 inches=0.9144 meter
foot-ft or '=12 inches, 0.333 yard=30.48 centimeters
inch-in or "=0.083 foot, 0.028 yard=2.54 centimeter

US-Metric Conversion: you will have word problems with conversions and will need to know this information.

Capacity
gallon-gal =4 quarts (231 cubic inches)=3.785 liters
quart-qt=2 pints (5=7.75 cubic inches)=0.946 liters
pint-pt=4 gills (28.875 cubic inches)=473.176 milliliters
pound-lb =12 ounces, 5760 grains=0.373 kilogram
ounce-oz=8 drams, 480 grains, 0.083 pound=31.103 grams
dram-dr =3 scruples, 60 grains=3.888 grams
bushel-bu=4 pecks (2150.42 cubic inches)=35.239 liters
peck-pk=8 quarts (537.605 cubic inches)=8.810 liters
cup-c.=8 ounces= 0.237 liters

Area
square mile-sq mi or mi2=640 acres, 102,400 square rods=2.590 square kilometers
acre -4840 square yards, 43,560 square feet,0.405 hectare,=4047 square meters
square rod-sq rd or rd2=30.25 square yards, 0.00625 acre=25.293 square meters
square yard-sq yd or yd2=1296 square inches, 9 square feet =0.836 square meter
square foot-sq ft or ft2=144 square inches, 0.111 square yard =0.093 square meter
square inch-sq in or in2=0.0069 square foot, 0.00077 square yard=6.452 square centimeters

Weight
pound-lb =16 ounces, 7000 grains=0.454 kilogram
ounce-oz=16 drams, 437.5 grains, 0.0625 pound=28.350 grams
short ton-20 short hundredweight, 2000 pounds=0.907 metric ton
long ton-20 long hundredweight, 2240 pounds=1.016 metric ton

Common nursing measurements in US and metric equivalents.
1 teaspoon (tsp)=1 fluid dram=5 mL (milliliters)
1 tablespoon(tbsp)=1/2 fluid oz.=15 mL (milliliters)
1 cup(c)=8 fluid oz.=240 mL(milliliters)
3 tsp. (tsp)=4 fluid drams=15 or 16 mL (milliliters)
1 gtt (drop)=1 minum=0.05 mL (milliliters)

General Math Facts: These are some of general facts that may be on the test.

Military Time: Is an unambiguous, concise method of expressing time used by the military, emergency services (law enforcement, firefighting, paramedics), hospitals, and other entities. **Example:** 5pm=1700 and 5am=0500

Units of time:
minute (1 min = 60 s)
hour (1 h = 60 min = 3.6 ks)
day (1 d = 24 h = 86.4 ks)
year (1 a = 365.25 d = 31.5576 Ms)
decade (10 years=3650 d)
century (100 a = 3.15576 Gs)
millennium (1000 years=1 ka = 31.5576 Gs)

Roman Numerals: Is the name for a number when it is written in the way the Romans used to write numbers.
I = 1
II = 2
III = 3
IV = 4

V =5
VI = 6
VII = 7
VIII = 8
IX = 9
X = 10
XI = 11
XV = 15
XVI = 16
XIX = 19
XX = 20

General Math Facts: These are some of general facts that will be on the test. Factors are either composite numbers or prime numbers (except that 0 and 1 are neither prime nor composite). The number 12 is a multiple of 3, because it can be divided evenly by 3.

3 x 4 = 12

3 and 4 are both factors of 12

12 is a multiple of both 3 and 4.

General Math Facts: These are some of general facts that will be on the test.

Number Square Cube

Number	Square	Cube
1	1	1
2	4	8
3	9	27
4	16	64
5	25	125
6	36	216
7	49	343
8	64	512
9	81	729
10	100	1000
11	121	1331
12	144	1728

General Math Facts: These are some of general facts that will be on the test. A common technique for remembering the order of operations is the abbreviation **"PEMDAS"**, which is turned into the phrase "Please Excuse My Dear Aunt Sally". It stands for "Parentheses, Exponents, Multiplication and Division, and Addition and Subtraction".

Example: 7 + (6 × 5sqrt + 3)

7 + (6 × 5sqrt + 3)

7 + (6 × 25 + 3) Start inside Parentheses, and then use Exponents First

7 + (150 + 3) Then Multiply

7 + (153) Then Add

7 + 153 Parentheses completed, last operation is an Add

160

Note: sqrt=means squared

Good Luck on your test!

9 SCIENCE-BIOLOGY

The Science portion of the HESI A2 test consists of three to four parts each part consists of 30 questions each: we will focus on Biology, Chemistry, and Anatomy & Physiology

Let's get started!

Biology: the scientific study of life

List in order the hierarchy system of biological organization 1-7.
1) Kingdom 2) Phylum 3) Class 4) Order 5) Family 6) Genus 7) Species

The smallest known microorganisms are: **Viruses**
Hypothesis: first step - statement /explanation of event
Experiment: 2nd step - repeatable procedure of gathering data to support hypothesis
Conclusion: last step to the scientific process

Water: covalent bond, polar - two hydrogens, one oxygen atom, important factors are polarity of hydrogen-oxygen bonds, high specific heat, the ability to stabilize climates, adhesion, freezing, and the ability to be a versatile solvent
What is the most important characteristic of water? Polarity of hydrogen-oxygen bonds

Hydrogen bonding: results in strong cohesive and adhesive properties

Specific heat: amount of heat needed to raise the temperature of 1 gram of a molecule by 1 degree C.

Cohesion: ability for molecule to stay bonded /attracted to same substance
Adhesion: sticks together

Carbohydrates: long chains, or polymers, of sugar. Carbohydrates provide a ready, easily used source of cellular fuel. The most important functions are storage, structure, and energy.
Proteins: The most significant contributor to cellular function. Organic compound containing nitrogen, carbon, hydrogen, and oxygen; building block of protein. Amino acids any of 20 basic building blocks of proteins - composed of a free amino (NH_2) end, a free carboxyl (COOH) end, and a side group (R).
Enzymes: proteins that control the various steps in all chemical reactions. a particular type of protein that acts as a catalyst for different reaction processes.
Nucleic acids: component of the molecules inheritance. Storing of genetic information. Deoxyribonucleic acid (DNA) is a unique molecule specific to a particular organism and contains the code that is necessary for replication. Ribonucleic acid (RNA) is used in transfer and as a messenger, in most species, or the genetic code.
DNA is double stranded and shaped like a double helix.

The sugar in DNA is__________. **Deoxyribose**
The sugar in RNA is_____. **Ribose**
What are the bases in DNA _____,_____,____,_____? **Adenine, Guanine, Thymine, Cytosine**
What are the bases in RNA___, _____, _____, _____? **Adenine, Guanine, Uracil, Cytosine**

Lipids: fats - fatty acids, phospholipids, steroids. Fatty acids grouped into two categories: saturated and unsaturated. Saturated fatty acids contain no double bonds in their hydrocarbon tail. These are solid, detrimental, and cause cardiovascular problems and are in diets that contain high quantities of saturated fats. Unsaturated fatty acids have one or more double bonds. These are liquid at room temperature.

Phospholipids: consist of two fatty acids of varying length bonded to a phosphate group. The phosphate group is charged and therefore polar, whereas the hydrocarbon tail of the fatty acids is nonpolar. This quality is important in the function of cellular membranes. The molecules combine in a way that creates a barrier that protects the cell.

Steroids: the last of the lipids. They are a component of membranes, but, more important, many are precursors to significant hormones. Group of chemical substances including certain hormones and cholesterol; they are fat soluble and contain little oxygen.

Metabolism: The sum of all chemical reactions that occur in an organism. In a cell, reactions take place in a series of steps called metabolic pathways, progressing from a standpoint of high energy to low energy. All of the reactions are catalyzed by the use of enzymes

Glucose Catabolism - Aerobic Respiration
• Cells generate ATP by cellular respiration.
• Aerobic respiration is the complete oxidation of glucose by glycolysis, the Krebs cycle, and the electron transport chain (ETC) and oxidative phosphorylation.
• The complete degradation of glucose by cellular respiration can be written:
C 6 H 12 O 6 + 6O 2 - 6CO 2 + 6H 2 O + Energy
• Glycolysis is connected to the Krebs cycle via a transitional step: the conversion of pyruvic acid (pyruvate) into Acetyl Coenzyme A (acetylCoA)
• Glycolysis occurs in the cytosol while the Krebs cycle and the ETC occur in the mitochondria.
Anaerobic Respiration
• Anaerobic respiration does not require oxygen.
• Glycolysis occurs, and may be followed by lactic acid fermentation, which is a way to continue glycolysis without the Krebs cycle or the ETC.

Cells: The fundamental unit of biology. There are two types of cells: prokaryotic and eukaryotic cells. Cells consist of many components, most of which are called organelles.

Prokaryotic Cells: Those containing no defined nucleus and a series of organelles that carry out the function of the cell as directed by the nucleus.
Eukaryotic Cells: Have a membrane-enclosed nucleus and a series of organelles that carry out the functions of the cell as directed by the nucleus. The eukaryotic cell is the more complex of the two cell types.
The plasma membrane of the eukaryotic cell determines selectively which substances can enter and leave the cell. Such a membrane is said to be? **Selectively permeable**

Nucleus: The first of the organelles is the nucleus, which contains the DNA of the cell in organized masses called chromosomes.

Chromosomes: Contain all the material for the regeneration of the cell as well as all instructions for the function of the cell. Every organism has a characteristic number of chromosomes specific to the particular species.

Ribosomes: Organelles that read the RNA produced in the nucleus and translate the gentic instructions to produce proteins. The two types of ribosomes aare interchangeable and have identical structures, although they have slightly different roles.
Ribosomes: Bound Ribosomes those found attached to the endoplasmic reticulum (ER). Free Ribosomes those found in the cytoplasm

Endoplasmic Reticulum: The ER is a membranous organelle found attached to the nuclear membrane and consists of two continuous parts. Through an electron microscope, part of the membranous system is covered with ribosomes. This section of the ER is referred to as rough ER. The other section of the ER lacks ribosomes and is referred to as smooth ER.

Rough ER: Responsible for protein synthesis and membrane production.

Smooth ER: It functions in detoxification and metabolism of multiple molecules

Lysosomes: Intracellular digestion takes place in lysosomes. Packed with hydrolytic enzymes, the lysosomes can hydrolyze proteins, fats, sugars, and nucleic acids.

Vacuoles: Membrane-enclosed structures that have various functions depending on cell type.

Cell Membrane: The most important component of the cell, contributing to protection, communication, and the passage of substances into and out of the cell. The cell membrane itself consists of a bilayer of phospholipids with proteins, cholesterol, and glycoproteins peppered throughout.

Mitochondria: Produce energy - found in eukaryotic cells and are the site of respiration. The powerhouse of a cell. (Organelles that produce cell energy.)
Which organelle is the synthesis of ATP associated? **Mitochondrion** makes ATP for energy
Chloroplasts in plants are the site for photosynthesis.

Glycolysis: the 1st step in cellular respiration conversion of glycogen to pyruvate, this takes place in cytosol and produces 2 molecules(m) of ATP, 2 m of pyruvate, and 2 m of NADH
The molecule that is used as the currency: ATP

Cellular Respiration: (catabolic pathways that lead to cellular energy production) Produces far more energy than does its anaerobic counterpart, fermentation. $C6H12O6 + 6O26CO2 + 6H2O$

Krebs cycle: Pyruvate transported into mitochondria creating cycles in matrix of mitochondria. Step two, the pyruvate is transported into a mitochondrion and used in the first of a series of reactions called the Krebs cycle. This cycle takes place in the matrix of the mitochondria, and for a single, consumed glucose molecule, two ATP molecules, six molecules of carbon dioxide, and six NADH molecules are produced.
Krebs cycle: The Krebs cycle which is also called the citric acid cycle, or the tricarboxylic acid (TCA) cycle is a group of 8 metabolic reactions that occur in the matrix of mitochondria. The first reaction of the cycle occurs when AcetylCoA reacts with oxaloacetic acid (OAA) in presence of water to form citric acid. In fact OAA combines with the acetyl group of AcetylCoa and water to form citric acid and Coenzyme A (CoA) is released. Since citric acid is the first intermediary, the cycle is often called citric acid cycle. The Krebs cycle is very important metabolically. The potential energy of glucose is removed step by step as redox reactions and decarboxylations remove all the carbons of glucose. The 2 pyruvic acids produced by glycolysis enter the cycle as 2 Acetyl CoA molecules. Each one produces:
• 2 molecules of C0 2
• 3 molecules of NADH + H +
• One molecule of ATP • one molecule of FADH 2
• By the end of the Krebs cycle all the potential energy of the original glucose has been extracted and is now under electron and proton form.
• Let us remember that glycolysis produced 2NADH + 2H + and that transformation of 2 pyruvic acids into AcetylCoA also produced 2NADH + 2H +.
• All these electron carriers will travel to the inner mitochondrial membrane to "dump" their electrons in the ETC.

Photosynthesis: Where energy originates; a precursor to the glucose molecule is produced in a process called photosynthesis. The chemical reaction representing this process is simply the reverse of cellular respiration. The only difference is the addition of light energy on the reactant side of the equation. Just as glucose is used to produce energy, so too must energy be used to produce glucose.
Photosynthesis Stage 1: Light Reactions
Those that convert solar energy to chemical energy. The cell accomplishes the production of ATP by absorbing light and using that energy to split a water molecule and transfer the electron, thus creating NADPH and producing ATP. These molecules are then used in the Calvin cycle to produce sugar.

Photosynthesis Stage 2: Calvin Cycle
The sugar produced is polymerized and stored as a polymer of glucose. These sugars are consumed by organisms or by the plant itself to produce energy by cellular respiration.

Cellular Reproduction: Cells reproduce by three different processes, all of which fall into two categories: sexual and asexual reproduction.

Asexual Reproduction: 1st Process of Cell Division: Binary Fission: In this process, the chromosome binds to the plasma membrane, where it replicates. Then as the cell grows, it pinches in two, producing two identical cells.

Asexual Reproduction:
Mitosis: This process of cell division occurs in five stages before pinching in two in a process called cytokinesis. The five stages are prophase, prometaphase, metaphase, anaphase, and telophase.
Prophase: The chromosomes are visibly separate, and each duplicated chromosome has two noticeable sister chromatids.
Prometaphase: The nuclear envelope begins to disappear, and the chromosomes begin to attach to the spindle that is forming along the axis of the cell.
Metaphase: With all the chromosomes aligning along what is called the metaphase plate, or the center of the cell.
Anaphase: Begins when chromosomes start to separate. In this phase the chromatids are considered separate chromosomes.
Telophase: The final phase. Here chromosomes gather on either side of the now separating cell. This is the end of mitosis.
Cytokinesis (2nd Process of cell division): The second process associated with cell division. During this phase, which is separate from the phases of mitosis, the cell pinches in two, forming two separate identical cells.

Sexual Reproduction: The offspring originates from a single cell, yielding all produced cells to be identical. In sexual reproduction, two cells contribute genetic material to the daughter cells, resulting in significantly greater variation. These two cells find and fertilize each other randomly, making it virtually impossible for cells to be alike.
Chromosome characteristics:
haploid (n) = one set of chromosomes
diploid (2n) = two sets of chromosomes
Eggs and sperm (gametes) are haploid
Diploid set for humans: 2n = 46

Meiosis: The process that determines how reproductive cells divide in a sexually reproducing organism. Meiosis consists of two distinct stages, meiosis one and meiosis two, resulting in four daughter cells. Each of these daughter cells contains half as many chromosomes as the parent. Preceding these events is a period called interphase.
Interphase: During interphase, the chromosomes are duplicated and the cell prepares for division.
1st Stage and 4 Phases of Meiosis: Prophase I, Metaphase I, Anaphase I, and Telophase I and Cytokinesis. The significant differences between Meiosis and Mitosis occur in Prophase I.
Prophase I: During this phase, nonsister chromatids of homologous chromosomes cross at numerous locations. Small sections of DNA are transferred between these chromosomes, resulting in increased genetic variation. The remaining three phases are the same as those in mitosis, with the exception that the chromosome pairs separate, not the chromosomes themselves. After the first cytokinesis, meiosis two begins. Here, all four stages identical to those of mitosis occur. The resulting four cells have half as many chromosomes as the parent cell.

Gregor Mendel: Discovered the basic principles of genetics. He determined that the observable traits in peas were passed from one generation to the next.

Alleles: For every trait expressed in a sexually reproducing organism, there are at least two alternative versions of a gene. For simple traits, the versions can be one of two types: dominant or recessive. Alleles are placed one per column for one gene and one per row for the other genes.
Homozygous: If both of the alleles are the same type, the organism is said to be homozygous for that trait.
Heterozygous: Alleles that are of different types.

HESI Hint: If an allele is dominant for a particular trait;, the letter chosen to represent that allele is capitalized. If the allele is recessive, then the letter is lowercased. If a dominant allele is present, then the phenotype expressed will be the dominant. The only way a recessive trait will be expressed is if both alleles are recessive.

Punnett Square: A device used to predict genotype (the combination of alleles) and phenotype (what traits will be expressed) of the offspring of sexual reproduction.

Pedigree: A family tree that traces the occurrence of a certain trait through several generations. A pedigree is useful in understanding the genetic past as well as the possible future.

Watson and Crick: They described DNA as a double helical structure that contains the four nitrogenous bases: adenine, thymine, guanine, and cytosine.

DNA Bonding Patterns: Each base forms hydrogen bonds with another base on the complementary strand. The bases have a specific bonding pattern. Adenine bonds with thymine and guanine bonds with cytosine. Because of this method of bonding, the strands can be replicated, producing identical strands of DNA. During replication, the strands are separated. Then, with the help of several enzymes, new complementary strands are created. This produces two new double=stranded segments of DNA identical to the original.
DNA Strand: Each gene along a strand of DNA is a template for protein synthesis. This production begins with a process called transcription.
Transcription: In this process an RNA strand, complementary to the original strand of DNA is produced. The piece of genetic material produced is called messenger RNA (mRNA)
RNA Strand: The RNA strand has nitrogenous bases identical to those in DNA with the exception of uracil, which is substituted for thymine.
mRNA: Functions as a messenger from the original DNA helix in the nucleus to the ribosomes in the cytosol or on the rough ER. Here, the ribosome acts as the site of translation. The mRNA slides through the ribosome. Every group of three bases along the stretch of RNA is called a codon, and each of these codes for specific amino acids.

Codon: Every group of three bases along the stretch of RNA.
AntiCodon: Located on a unit called transfer RNA (tRNA), which carries a specific amino acid. It binds to the ribosome when its codon is sliding through the ribosome
Stop Codon: Stop point of amino acids chain. The chain is released into the cytoplasm and the protein folds onto itself and forms its complete conformation.
Which movement requires carrier protein but no direct cellular energy? **Facilitated transport**
The movement of substances from lesser concentration to higher concentration is called? **Active transport**

Deposition: Gas to Solid Passage of water through the membrane of a cell is called? **Osmosis.** Also allows nutrients, gases, and molecules to enter and leave cell.
During the process of diffusion molecules moves from a region of high concentration to one of low concentration. Molecule is dissolved in water to pass through the cell membrane.
Keratin is a fibrous protein in hair, fingernails, horns, reptilian scales, and feathers.
Collagen the protein that gives shape to the skin, tendons, ligaments, cartilage, and bones of animals

Microscope: The most careful and exacting observations awaited the simple single-lens microscope hand-fashioned by Antonie van Leeuwenhoek, a Dutch linen merchant and self-made microbiologist.

10 SCIENCE-CHEMISTRY

Chemistry: 3 States of Matter: Solid, Liquid, Gas

Solid: A solid is matter that has definite shape and volume.
Liquid & Gas: Matter that is fluid and takes the shape of its container. Unlike solids and liquids, the volume of gases will change drastically with changes in temperature and pressure.

Vaporization: Liquid to Gas
Condensation: Gas to Liquid
Melting: Solid to Liquid
Freezing: Liquid to Solid
Sublimation: Solid to Gas

Freezing point of water F: 32
Boiling point of water F: 212
Freezing point of water C: 0
Boiling point of Water C: 100
Freezing point of water K: 273
Boiling point of Water K: 373

Homogeneous Mixture: Mixture with uniform density throughout and no distinguishable components.
Heterogeneous Mixture: Mixture in which the components are readily distinguished.

Elements: substances that exist in the simplest form and are represented by a specific letter or combinations of letters.
Compounds: Combinations of elements in whole number ratios.

Chemical Equations: is a symbolic representation of a chemical reaction in terms of chemical formulas.

Reactants: Ingredients that react to produce a desired result called products. Equations are written in the following manner:
Reactants -- Products

The Law of Conservation of Mass: States that mass cannot be created or destroyed during a chemical reaction. Therefore, once the reactants have been written and the products predicted, the equation must be balanced. The same number of each element must be represented on both sides of the equation.

Chemical Reactions: The breaking of bonds and the reforming of new bonds to create new chemical compounds with different chemical formulas and different chemical properties.
5 Main Types of Chemical Reactions:
Synthesis, Decomposition, Combustion, Single Replacement, and Double Replacement
Synthesis Reaction: Two elements combine to form a product.
Decomposition Reaction: The breaking of a compound into component parts.
Combustion Reaction: The reaction of a compound or element with oxygen. In the combustion of a hydrocarbon, the products are CO_2 and H_2O
$CH_4 + 2O_2 \rightarrow CO_2 + 2H_2O$
Replacement Reaction: Involve ionic compounds and whether the reaction will take place is based on the activity of the metals involved.
Single Replacement Reaction: Consist of a more active metal reacting with an ionic compound containing a less active metal to produce a new compound. $Mg(s) + 2 HCl(aq) \rightarrow MgCl_2(aq) + H_2(g)$

Double Replacement Reaction: Involve two ionic compounds. The positive ion from one compound combines with the negative ion of the other compound. The result is two new ionic compounds that have "switched partners."
$KOH + H_2SO_4 ---> K_2SO_4 + H_2O$

Atomic Number: Represents the number of protons a given element contains.
Atomic Mass: An average of the masses of each of its isotopes as they occur in nature. By subtracting the atomic number from the mass number of an element, it is possible to calculate the number of neutrons contained by a given isotope of a certain element.

Period Table Columns and Rows: The groups (columns) and periods (rows) are significant. It is possible to predict with accuracy the charge of an atom of certain elements when as an ion dissolved in solution or as an ion in a compound based on its location on the periodic table.
1. Groups are columns.
2. Periods are rows.
Group 1A, 2A, 3A have what charges? +1, +2, +3
Group 4A, 5A, 6A, 7 have what charges? -4, -3, -2, -1
Group VlllA is what group and what charge? Noble Gases, no charge, neutral

Atomic Structure: The atom consists of three component parts: Protons, Neutrons, and Electrons.
Protons: Have a positive charge
Electrons: Have a negative charge
Neutrons: Have no charge
Protons have the same what? **Mass**
Relative to the proton, what's the difference in mass of electron? **1840 times less**
The number of protons in an element is the what? **Atomic number**
The sum of protons and neutrons in an atom is called? **Mass number**
The majority of the volume of an atom is? **Empty space**

HESI HINT: nucleus contains the protons and neutrons, electrons are in orbital clouds.

The majority of the volume of an atom is? **Empty space**
In chemical reactions, atoms try to reach stable what? **Electron configurations**

Molecules: A group of two or more atoms linked together by sharing electrons in a chemical bond. Molecules are the fundamental components of chemical compounds and are the smallest part of a compound that can participate in a chemical reaction.
Isotope: Atoms with the same number of protons but different numbers of neutrons.
Ions: electrically charged atoms.
Anion: An ion with a negative charge.
Cation: An ion with a positive charge

Nuclear reactions: Are those that take place in the nucleus, to obtain stable nuclear configurations
Radioactivity: word used to describe the emission of particles from an unstable nucleus
What are the 3 types of radiation? Are the particles that are emitted: **alpha, beta, and gamma.**
Alpha radiation: Emission of helium ions. These particles contain 2 protons and 2 neutrons, causing them to have a charge of +2. It is common to omit the fact that these particles are charged.
Penetration from alpha particles can be stopped by? A piece of paper
What is beta radiation composed of? Product of the decomposition of a neutron
high-energy, high-speed electrons. These particles are negatively and have no mass
Gamma radiation: high-energy electromagnetic radiation
Gamma radiation lacks? **Charge and mass**
Gamma radiation can be stopped by? Several feet of concrete or several inches of lead

Two types of chemical bonding? **Covalent and ionic**
Ionic bond is generally between what? Electrostatic attraction between 2 oppositely charged ions
Single covalent bond: formed when 2 atoms share a pair of electrons
Double covalent bond: formed when 2 electron pairs are shared
Triple covalent bond: formed when 3 electron pairs are shared
What is the strongest of any type of chemical bond? Covalent bond.
Covalent bond: When nonmetal elements bond, they share electrons between each other. This sharing is called a covalent bond.
If not all elements share electrons equally within a covalent bond what occurs? A nonpolar covalent bond results when the shared electrons orbit both atoms equally. An example of a nonpolar bond is hydrogen gas.
Polarity is based on?   The difference in electronegativity values for the elements involved in the bond
The greater the difference in electronegativity the more polar the bond will be.

Intermolecular forces: a type of attraction between particles.
These forces are:
1. Hydrogen bonding
2. Dipole interactions
3. Dispersion forces

What the strongest of the intermolecular forces? **Hydrogen bonding**
1. This attraction is considered weak
2. This attraction is the weakest
1. Dipole interactions
2. Dispersion

Van der Waals forces: dipole and dispersion

Hydrogen bonds: attraction for a hydrogen atom by a highly electronegative element
What elements are generally involved in hydrogen bonds?   **Fluorine, Chlorine, Oxygen and Nitrogen**

Dipole Interactions: The attractions of one dipole for another. Created when an electron pair in a covalent bond is shared unequally. The result is a bond in which the more highly electronegative element is slightly negative and the less electronegative element is slightly positive. The positive end of a dipole in one compound will be attracted to the negative end of another dipole in a separate compound. This attraction is considered a weak intermolecular force.

Dispersion Forces: The weakest of all intermolecular forces. Moving electrons within an element or compound concentrate themselves on one side of an atom. This causes a momentary dipole, which would be attracted to another momentary dipole in an adjoining element or compound. Usually found in nonpolar covalent compounds.
Mole: The amount of a substance that contains $6.02 \times 10(23)$ representative particles of that substance. A mole of a substance is the same as its atomic mass. **True.**
Solution: is a homogenous mixture that combines a solute and a solvent
Solute: is the substance that dissolved in the solvent
Molarity: moles of solute/liters of solution.

Stoichiometry: The part of chemistry that deals with the quantities and the numeric relationship between compounds in a chemical reaction.
Example: A piece of metallic iron (10moles) was dissolved in conc. HCl. The reaction formed H_2 and $FeCl_2$.
a) Balance: $Fe+HCl>FeCl_2+H_2$ and determine
b) Amount of formed $FeCl_2$
c) Amount of used HCl
The solution
a) $Fe + 2HCl = FeCl_2+H_2$
b) As we can see from the balanced equation (a) n (Fe) = n ($FeCl_2$), 10 moles of $FeCl_2$ was formed in the reaction.
c) The balanced equation (a) tells us that n (HCl) = 2n (Fe) --> 20 moles of HCl was used.

Equilibrium: not all chemical reactions proceed to completion; some simply slow down, with leftover amounts of reactant still present. These types of reactions said to be at equilibrium. At this point, reactants forming products at the same rate that products are forming reactants. The reactions is said to be reversible.

Four Ways to Increase Reaction Rate:
Increase the Temperature; Increase the Surface Area, Increase the Concentrations of Reactants, Or Add a Catalyst.
TEMPERATURE: increasing---causes particles 2 have greater kinetic energy
SURFACE AREA: Increasing---gives particles more opportunity 2 come in contact
CONCENTRATION: When increased rate of reaction accelerate, decreased rate is reduced
CATALYST: Accelerates reaction by reducing activation energy
When the concentration is increased, the rate of the reaction is ___________. **accelerated**
When concentration is decreased, the rate of the reaction is __________.   **reduced**
Catalyst: accelerates a reaction by reducing the activation energy, or the amount of energy necessary for a reaction to occur. Is the catalysts used up in the reaction? No, and it can be collected at reaction completion

Oxidation: is the removal of electrons from a molecule.
Reduction: is the gain of electrons by a molecule.
Rules for determining oxidation state:
1. Elemental atoms have an oxidation number of zero.
2. The oxidation number of any simple ion is the charge of the ion.
3. The oxidation number for oxygen in compound is always -2.
4. The oxidation number for hydrogen in compound is +1.
5. The sum of the oxidation numbers equals the charge on the molecule or polyatomic ions.
Oxidation example: After electrons were discovered, chemists became convinced that oxidation-reduction reactions involved the transfer of electrons from one atom to another. From this perspective, the reaction between magnesium and oxygen is written as follows. $2 Mg + O_2 ----> 2 [Mg^{2+}][O^{2-}]$
In the course of this reaction, each magnesium atom loses two electrons to form an Mg^{2+} ion. $Mg ----> Mg^{2+} + 2 e-$
And, each O_2 molecule gains four electrons to form a pair of O^{2-} ions. $O_2 + 4 e- ----> 2 O^{2-}$
Because electrons are neither created nor destroyed in a chemical reaction, oxidation and reduction are linked.

Acid-Base: is known also pH.
pH low: acidic
pH high: basic
Acid: SOUR / TART, formulas begin with H , conduct electrical current; pH less than 7
Base: BITTER, produce OH, feels slippery; pH greater than 7
Neutralization: Process which occurs when an acid and a base react to produce a salt and water. The result is a pH near 7.

HESI Hint: By manipulation of the quantity of acid and/or base in a solution, the pH can be altered. The process of neutralization occurs when an acid and a base react to produce a salt and water. Generally, this results in a neutral pH or pH close to 7.

Notes:

11 SCIENCE-ANATOMY & PHYSIOLOGY

Anatomy and Physiology: Directional terms
1. Superior: toward head
2. Inferior: toward feet
3. Proximal: close to point of origin
4. Distal: away from point of origin
5. Medial: close to midline of body
6. Lateral: away from midline of body
7. Ipsilateral: on same side of body
8. Contralateral: on opposite side of body
9. Bilateral: two of the same (eyes, ears, hands,)
10. Dorsal/Posterior: back of the body
11. Ventral/Anterior: front of body

Planes/Section:
1. Sagittal sections: divide body into right and left halves
a.midsagittal: equal halves b. parasagittal: unequal halves
2. Horizontal section: divides body into upper and lower halves
3. Frontal sections: divides body into front and back halves

Dorsal Cavity:
Cranial cavity
Spinal cavity

Ventral Cavity:
The orbits and the nasal cavities
Oral cavity
Thoracic cavity
Abdominopelvic cavity

Tissue: group of similar cells
Four Fundamental Tissues: Epithelial, Connective, Nerve, Muscle

Epithelial tissue: Characteristics:
Cells tightly packed
Very little intercellular space
Cells rest on a basement membrane
Relatively avascular
Function: as covering or lining

Squamous epithelium: Flat, scale like cells
Cuboidal cells: cells with almost same height/width
Columnar cells: cells that is taller than they are wide

Simple epithelium: One layer of cells
Found in part of body not subjected to much wear/tear

Stratified epithelium: Many layer of cells

Found in parts of body subjected to much wear/tear
Skin: stratified squamous epithelium

Oral epithelium: stratified squamous epithelium (nonkeratinized - moist)
Pseudostratified epithelium: has one layer of cells but gives a false appearance of being many layered due to unequal heights of the cells

Transitional epithelium: made of cells capable of changing shape , found within urinary bladder, gives bladder capacity to stretch

Connective tissue:
Loose connective tissue: made of cells called fibroblasts. Forms scar tissue. Most abundant in body. Dense connective tissue: protein fibers better organized
Example:
Tendon - connect muscle to bone
Ligament - connect bone to bone
Function: forms supportive frame work of body

Connective tissue:
Cartilage: Made of cells called Chondrocytes
Does not have good blood supply - poor healing Adipose tissue - fat tissue and made of cells called Adipocytes. They are capable of storing fat.
Function: Conserve heat, protective padding for internal organs
Blood / vascular connective tissue
Have blood cells which include red blood cell, white blood cell, platelet
Intercellular substances- liquid called plasma

Connective tissue:
Membrane: Made of epithelial and connective tissue
Mucus membrane: line structures that open to the outside
Serous membrane: around internal organs
Pericardium - heart
Pleura- lung
Peritoneum- abdominal organs
Synovial membrane- around joints

Nerve tissue: Made of nerve cells or neurons, can generate and conduct nerve signals

Muscle tissue: Made of muscle cells. Specialized tissue for contraction / relaxation. Skeletal muscle tissue-attached to bone voluntary and striated. Cardiac tissue - muscle of heart. Involuntary, Striated, and branched. Smooth muscle-Involuntary, nonstriated, found in all hollow, internal organs.

What is a cell? The basic unit of life and the building block of tissues and organs.
What is an organelle? A object inside a cell that has a specific function.
What is a nucleus? Contains deoxyribonucleic acid (DNA). Main part of a Eukaryotic cell.
What is a Ribosome? Used for synthesis of proteins.
What are enzymes? Proteins (99%) that regulate all chemical reactions in the body.
What is Mitosis necessary for? Growth and repair.
What happens during Mitosis? The DNA is duplicated and distributed evenly to two daughter cells.
What is Meiosis? Special cell division that takes place in the gonads (ovaries and testes), the chromosome number is reduced from 46 to 23, so when the egg and sperm unite in fertilization the zygote will have the correct number of chromosomes.

What are the principal membranes? Mucous, serous, synovial, and cutaneous - composed of epithelial tissue.

What are the different types of glands? Sudoriferous, sebaceous, and ceruminous.
Where does cartilage replace bone in embryonic development? Joints, the thorax, and various rigid tubes.
What is the largest organ in the body? The skin.
Function: Protection, Excretion of wastes - sweat, Regulation of body temperature - sweat, Sensation, Absorption, Immunity, Reservoir of blood
What does the skin consist of? Two layers: the epidermis (the outer most protective layer of dead keratinized epithelial cells; and the dermis which is the underlying layer of connective tissue with blood vessels, nerve endings, and the associated skin structures.

What are the layers of the Epidermis?
1. Stratum basale - made of cells that are in a constant state of mitosis
2. Stratum spinosum - cells in this layer have spinous processes
3. Stratum granulosum - cells in this layer have keratohyalin granules which later becomes keratin - a substance that waterproofs the skin
4. Stratum lucidum - found only in thick skin - in palms and soles of feet . This layer has cells that contain eleidin granules that gives skin a translucent appearance
5. Outer most layer - Stratum corneum - has dead cells that are constantly being shed

What layer does mitosis occurs in the Epidermis? Stratum basale

What is Melanin? A protein pigment found in epidermal cells; protect skin against radiation from the sun

What does the Dermis contain? Fibrous connective tissue with blood vessels, sensory nerve endings, hair follicles, and glands.
What are the two types of sweat glands? **Eccrine and Apocrine.**
What do Sebaceous glands release? **Sebum**
What is oil produced by? - Through the hair follicle that lubricates the skin and prevents drying.
Holocrine secretion, in which whole cells of the gland are part of the secretion.

What are the appendages of the skin? Hair and nails.
What are hair and nails composed of? A strong protein called keratin.
What can hair, skin and nails be used for in diagnosis? They may show changes in different diseases that can be used in clinical conditions. i.e., skin cancer is a clinical condition that is associated with the skin.
What does the body's framework consist of? Bone, cartilage, ligaments, plus the joints between the bones.

Skeletal system: Skeletal system has 206 bones

HESI hint: Please review all bones especially the ones in the feet, ankle, and toes.

What are the functions of the skeletal system? Supportive framework, movement, storage of calcium, bone marrow-red and yellow
What are the different shapes of bones? Long, short, flat, irregular, and sesamoid.

Bone: made of bone cells
Osteoprogenitor cells- parent cells that form osteoblast
Osteoblast- bone forming cells
Osteocyte - mature osteoblasts, perform everyday function of bone
Osteoclast- bone eroding /destroying cell

Skeletal system:
The axial skeleton consist of 28 bones in the skull.

Upper Portion of Appendicular skeleton consists of:
Pectoral/shoulder girdle
Clavicle
Scapula

Upper extremity (arm/hand)

Bones of the Arm (Upper Extremity)
Humerus
Radius
Ulna
Carpals (wrist bones)
Metacarpals (bones of hand)
Phalanges (14 bones of the fingers)

Lower Portion of the Appendicular skeleton consists of:
Pelvic girdle/os coxae
Bones of lower extremity (leg/feet)

Os Coxae consists of:
A fused ilium
Ischium
Pubis

Bones of the Lower Extremity:
Femur (thighbone)
Tibia
Fibula
Tarsals (ankle bones)
Metatarsals (bones of the foot)
Phalanges (14 toe bones)

Joints:
With space - synovial joint
Without space- Fibrous joint- fibrous tissue fills up joint space
Cartilaginous joint- cartilage fills up joint space

Joints: Functional classification
Synarthroses -do not allow any movement ex. Sutures gomphosis (joint between teeth and bone)
Amphiathroses - allow minimal movement ex. Pubic symphathses
Diarthroses - allow wide range of movement ex. Synovial joint

Synovial joint - classification: Based on shape of bone that forms the joint ball and socket joint - ball like surface of 1 bone fit into cuplike surface of another bone ex hip joint and shoulder joint
Hinge joint - convex surface of 1 bone fits into concave surface of another bone ex. Elbow joint, knee joint
Pivot joint - peg like surface of 1 bone fits into ring like surface of another bone ex. between atlas and axis
Gliding joint - flat surface of 2 bones glide over 1 another. Ex- between tarsal bones
Ellipsoidal joint- is a biaxial joint in which two principal axes of motion are at right angles to each other. Ex. the wrist joint
Saddle joint- It allows movement in two directions. The saddle joint gives the human thumb the ability to "crossover" the palm of the hand.

Movement possible at synovial joint:
1. **Flexion** - decreases in angle between articulating bones
2. **Extension** - increases in angle between articulating bones
3. **Abduction** - move away from body
4. **Adduction** - move toward from body
5. **Pronation**- palms face downwards@ elbow

6. **Supination** - palms face upwards @ elbow
7. **Inversion** - sole faces medially@ ankle joint
8. **Eversion** - sole face laterally
9. **Depression** -lower mandible (open mouth) temporo mandible
10. **Elevation**- elevate mandible (close mouth) temporo mandible

How to muscles produce movement?
1. They contract in response to nervous stimulation
2. Myosin and actin filaments within the muscle cell/fiber slide together
What do muscle cells consist of? **Cell membrane - sarcolemma**

Cytoplasm - sarcoplasm
Endoplasmic reticulum - sarcoplasmic reticulum
Transverse (T) :Tubules - communicating channels
Myofilaments- protein fibers that give muscle cells ability to contract/relax
What two things must be present in order for a muscle cell to contract? Calcium and ATP (Adenosine triphosphate)

How do muscles produce movement? When muscle receives nerve signal to contract Ca+ ions are released from endoplasmic reticulum
Ca+ ions remove the troponin-tropomyosin complex exposing the myosin binding sites
The filaments slide over one another
Muscle shortens and contracts
When nerve signal stops the filaments slide away from each other and muscle returns to original position.

Muscles can be classified by movements:
Antagonist- Produces the opposite movement of a prime mover
Synergists- A muscle that may work in cooperation with a prime mover
Flexor Muscles- Reduce the angle at the joint
Extensors- Increase the angle at the joint
Abductors- Draw a limb away from the midline
Adductors- Return the limb back toward the body

Nervous System:
Central nervous system (CNS) - brain and spinal cord
Peripheral nervous system (PNS) - all nerves that leave brain and spinal cord

Nervous System: function
Control / regulate all body activities by generating nerve signal
They have 3 stages
1. Receives stimuli
2. Interpret the stimuli
3. Respond to the stimuli

Neurons: performs as all the functions of nervous system. Hence referred to as functional unit of NS
Neurons parts:
Cell body
Axon
Dendrite
Myelin sheath (insulation)

Peripheral nervous system (PNS): Afferent nervous system - include all nerves that go to brain and spinal cord (sensory)

Efferent nervous system - include all nerves that leave brain and spinal cord (motor)
What do Sensory (Afferent) neurons transmit? Motor neurons carry impulses from the CNS to effector organs

What do Motor (Efferent) neurons transmit? Sensory neurons carry electrical signals (impulses) from receptors or sense organs to the CNS

Efferent nervous system: Somatic nervous system- includes nerves leave brain and spinal cord and go to skeletal muscle.

Autonomic nerves system: (ANS) includes nerves that leave brain and spinal cord and go to smooth muscle, cardiac muscle and glands. Sympathetic-flight or fight response and Parasympathetic-rest and relax such as digestion

Brain: Cerebrum-sensory and movement
Cerebellum--Coordination of movement
Hypothalamus-Coordinates activities of both nervous and endocrine system "thermostat" of body - regulates body temperature. Also has hunger, thirst and satiety center
Thalamus-Collection of nerve cell bodies above midbrain
Function: serves as an interpretation center for pain and temperature sensation.
Midbrain (brainstem)-responsible for movement of head / neck in response
Pons (brainstem)-midsection -has breathing centers - apneustic center and pneumotaxic center
Medulla oblongata (brainstem)-control heart rate, breathing and BP

Spinal Cord: serves as a pathway for messages traveling to and from brain
Serves as an interpretation center for some reflexes
Nerves that come out of spinal cord
They are 31 pairs
Neck - cervical - 8
Chest - thoracic - 12 Abdomen - lumbar - 5
Pelvis - sacral - 5 and cocygeal - 1
Called mixed nerves: have both sensory and motor component

When spinal nerves leave the vertebral canal - they divide into 2 branches
Anterior - ventral rami (branch)
Posterior - dorsal rami

Endocrine system: The endocrine system is a collection of glands that produces hormones, which are necessary for normal bodily functions. The hormones regulate metabolism, growth and sexual development. These glands release the hormones directly into the bloodstream, where they are transported to organs and tissues throughout the entire body.
Endocrine glands: Ductless glands. Produce hormones (emptied into bloodstream)
Head
Hypothalamus
Pituitary gland
Pineal gland
Neck
Thyroid gland
Parathyroid gland
Chest
Thymus gland
Abdomen
Pancreas
Adrenal gland
Pelvis
Testes
Ovaries

Hypothalamus: neuroendocrine structure produces regulatory hormones that control the pituitary gland.

Pituitary gland: Known as master gland. Because it controls the secretion of hormones. The pituitary gland constantly monitors body functions and sends signals to remote organs and glands to control their function and maintain the appropriate environment.

Pituitary gland: Anterior lobe hormones-Tropic hormones
GH - growth hormones
Facilitates growth and development
MSH - melanocyte stimulating hormones
Stimulates melanocytes on skin
FSH - follicle stimulating hormones
Stimulate testes / ovaries to produce sperms/eggs
LH - lutenizing hormones
Stimulate testes/ovaries to produce testosterone/ estrogen and progesterone
TSH - thyroid stimulating hormone- stimulates thyroid gland to make its hormones
ACTH - adreno cortico trophic hormone - stimulates adrenal gland to make its hormones
PRL - prolactin - stimulates mammary gland for lactation
Pituitary gland: Posterior lobe hormones
ADH - antiduritic hormone - act on DCT of nephrons to reabsorb water from filtrate
OT - oxytocin - act on pregnant uterus to induce labor

Cardiovascular system - Blood
Physical characteristic of blood (about 5- 6 liters)
- Red blood
- Thicker than water
- Warm
- Salty
- pH neutral

Blood - composition (When we centrifuge the blood)
1. Liquid component
- Plasma
2. Cellular component
- RBCs-(red blood cells)-erythrocytes
- WBCs-(white blood cells)-leukocytes
- Platelets-thrombocytes

Cardiovascular system – Blood- Functions: -
Transportation
1. Nutrients
2. Wastes
3. Oxygen
4. Co2
5. Hormones
Regulation
1. Blood pressure
2. pH
3. Temperature
Protection
1. Against infection
2. Blood loss

Cardiovascular system - Blood
RBCs- most numerous of blood cells
- About 5 million in number
- Do not have nucleus

- Appear as biconcave disks
- Have red pigment called hemoglobin
- Strong affinity for O2
- Life span 120 days
- Old RBCs destroyed in spleen
-Transport O2
-Gives blood its color

Cardiovascular system - Blood
WBCs-largest of the 3 blood cells
- Have nucleus
- Nucleus may / may not be lobed
- Cytoplasm may / may not have granules
- Life span - few hours to few days
- 5 different types

Neutrophil:
Nucleus has 2 - 6 lobes
Cytoplasm has fine pink granules
Function: involved in acute inflammation

Eosinophil:
Nucleus has 2 lobes
Cytoplasm has coarse pink granules
Function: involved in allergic reaction

Basophil:
Nucleus has 2 lobes
Cytoplasm has blue / black granules
Granules obscure nucleus
Function: causes hypersensitivities

Lymphocyte:
Nucleus has no lobes
Cytoplasm has no granules
Nucleus fills up entire cell
Function: provide immunity

Monocyte:
Nucleus has no lobes
Cytoplasm has no granules
Nucleus maybe bean shaped
Function: involved in chronic infection

Cardiovascular system - Blood
Platelets /Thrombocytes (small blue dot)
Fragments of a large cell called megakaryocyte
About 250,000 to 400,000 in number
Life span 4 to 10 days
Function: involved in the blood clotting mechanism

Cardiovascular system – Heart: Is a muscular organ about the size of a fist, located just behind and slightly left of the breastbone. The heart pumps blood through the network of arteries and veins called the cardiovascular system.

Wall - heart - layers
Outer - epicardium - connective tissue
Middle - myocardium - cardiac muscle
Inner - endocardium - epithelial tissue

Chambers of heart - 4
Upper 2 - atria (receiving chambers)
Lower 2 - ventricles (output chambers)
Right side of heart separated from left side of heart to prevent mixing of oxygenated blood (L.side) with deoxygenated blood (R.side)

Cardiovascular system - Heart
Left ventricle LV thickest wall
Heart valves (4)
2 atrioventricular valve (AV valves)
2 semilunar valves

Atrioventricular valves:
Bicuspid /mitral valve - between LA and LV
Tricuspid valve - between RA and RV
Chordae tendinae and papillary muscle are regulate opening and closing of AV valves
Semilunar valves (2)
1. Pulmonary semilunar valve between RV and pulmonary artery
2. Aortic semilunar valve between LV and aorta

Autorhythmicity: ability to set its own pace due to presence of specialized tissue called conduction system

Conduction system Include:
- Sinoatrial node (SA node) pace maker of the heart
- Atrioventricular node (AV node)
- Bundle of His
- Purkinje fiber

Cardiovascular system - Heart
EKG/ECG: (electrocardiogram) is an electrical recording of the heart and is used in the investigation of heart disease
ECG: recording of heart
P wave: atrial systole
QRS complex: ventricular systole
T wave: ventricular diastole

Cardiovascular system - Heart
Cardiac cycle
1st half: atrial systole, ventricular diastole
2nd half: ventricular systole, atrial diastole

Artery
1. Transports oxygenated blood (exception: pulmonary artery)
2. Always transport blood away from heart
3. Deeper in location
4. Thicker wall
5. Do not have valves
6. Pulsations felt
7. Used to check pulse, BP

Vein
1. Transport deoxygenated blood (exception: pulmonary veins)
2. Always transport blood towards heart
3. Superficial in location
4. Thin wall
5. Have valves
6. No pulsations felt
7. Used to obtain blood samples and for transfusions (infusion- IVs)

Cardiovascular system - Heart
What are the smallest arteries called? **Arterioles**
What are the Superior and Inferior Vena Cavae? Large veins that empty into the right atrium of the heart.

HESI hint: Review the major arteries and veins of the body.

Respiratory system:
Involved in respiration. Exchange of respiratory gases (O_2, CO_2) between atmosphere, lung, blood and body cells.
Respiration: happens in 3 stages
1. Pulmonary ventilation - gas exchange between atmosphere and lung
2. External respiration: gas exchange between lung and blood
3. Internal respiration: gas exchange between blood and body cells.

Respiratory system: include
Nose
Pharynx
Larynx
Trachea
Bronchi
Lung

Lungs:
R. lung
(3 lobes) - Superior - Middle - Inferior
(2 fissures) - Oblique, horizontal- No cardiac notch
L. lung
(2 lobes) superior- inferior
(1 fissure)
Oblique-has cardiac notch
Lungs: Each lung has millions of air sacs called alveoli
Alveoli: kept open by special substances called surfactant

Lungs
Physiology of respiration
Gas exchanges take place along a pressure gradient (from high to low) O_2 →from atmospheres CO_2 →metabolic waste produces by body cells
Lungs
Atmosphere → lung blood →body cell
Breathe in →O_2 → O_2 → O_2
Breathe out →CO_2 → CO_2 →CO_2

Digestive system:
Involved digestion
Digestion: breakdown of food so it can be easily absorbed into blood stream.

Chemical: breakdown food using digestive enzymes
Mechanical: breakdown food by mechanical action ex; chewing

Digestive system:
Main organs
- Mouth
- Esophagus
- Stomach
- Small intestine
- Large intestine
- Rectum
- Anal canal (Anus)
Accessory structures:
- Liver
- Gallbladder
- Salivary glands

Digestive system:
Saliva
- Predominantly water
- Contains digestive enzyme
- Salivary amylase or ptyalin (ptyalin breakdown starch)
Salivary glands:
3 pairs (exocrine gland)
1. Parotid gland - (Stensens duct)
2. Submandibular gland (Wharton's duct)
3. Sublingual gland - (ducts of Rivini)

Digestive system:
In mouth
- Mechanical and chemical digestion of starch and sugar
- Only mechanical digestion of proteins and lipids
- Semi solid food that is swallowed is called Bolus
Most organs involved in digestion located in abdominal cavity surrounded by Peritoneum
Digestive tract wall - layers (4)
- Inner mucosa - epithelium tissue
- Sub mucosa - connective tissue
- Muscularis - smooth muscle tissue
- Outer - serosa - connective tissue

Digestive system:
Esophagus:
- Narrow tube that connects pharynx to stomach
- Extends through neck, thoracic cavity, passes through diaphragm to enter stomach in abdominal cavity
Mucosa
Submucosa
Muscularis
Serosa
Merely transports food down into stomach

Digestive system:
Gastric glands:
1. Chief/Zymogenic cells - produce pepsinogen

2. Parietal/Oxyntic cell - produce HCL
3. Mucus cell - produce mucus
4. Enteroendocrine cell - produce hormone called gastrin
Physiology:
Digestion of starch continues with help of salivary amylase
- Digestion of protein begin
- No enzyme to digest fat
- Semiliquid food that moves from stomach to small intestine is called chyme

Digestive system:
Small intestine: Digestion is completed and all food and water absorbed into bloodstream from here. Small intestine has 3 parts.
1. Duodenum - 1st
2. Jejunum - middle section
3. Ileum - terminal section
- Mucosa - has intestinal glands/ crypts of Lieberkuln
- Submucosa - has folds called "villi" and increase surface area for food absorption
- Muscularis
- Serosa

Digestive system:
Digestive enzymes: from pancreas and liver are brought by ducts to small intestine to complete digestion
Physiology:
Carbohydrates → digested to →glucose
Protein →digested to→ amino acids absorbed into blood stream
Lipids →digested to →glycerol and fatty acids

Digestive system:
Large intestine/ colon: Unique land marks
The ascending colon, the transverse colon, the descending colon, the sigmoid colon and the rectum.
Haustra - pouches
Taenia coli - 3 longitudinal muscle bands
Function:
- Formation of stools
- Normal bacteria that reside in colon ferment food and produce gas

Digestive system:
Pancreas: - leaf, shaped gland close to duodenum- even through food does not pass through this structure it makes all 3 digestive enzymes
Pancreatic juice
1. Pancreatic amylase - digests starch
2. Trypsin and Chymotrypsin - break down protein
3. Pancreatic lipase - break down lipids

Digestive system:
Liver
Second largest organ in the body
- made of cells hepatocytes (produce bile)
Bile: Necessary for emulsification of fat
Emulsification prepare fats for action by pancreatic lipase

Digestive system:
Anus: used primarily for the dispensing of fecal matter

Urinary system:
Includes:
kidneys
ureter
urinary bladder
urethra
These organs control the amount of water and salts that are absorbed back into the blood and what is taken out as waste. This system also acts as a filtering mechanism for the blood.

Urinary system:
Kidney
1. Regulate volume, composition, and PH of blood
2. Produce a substance called renin which is involved in regulating BP
3. Produce a hormone called erythropoietin
Erythropoietin stimulates bone marrow to produce RBCs Location
- Abdominal cavity
- Behind peritoneum - retroperitoneal organ

Urinary system:
Nephron: perform all the function of kidney, hence referred to as functional units of kidney
Nephron - parts
- Glomerulus
- Bowman's capsules
Forms renal corpuscle
- Proximal convoluted tubule (PCT)
- Loop of Henle
- Distal convoluted tubule (DCT)
- Collecting tubule (CT)
Nephrons filter blood and remove wastes
Nephrons perform this function by forming urine

Urinary system:
Forming urine has 3 steps
1. Glomerular filtration
2. Tubular reabsorption
3. Tubular secretion
Glomerular filteration
- Glomerulus - only part of nephron that has blood capillaries
- Bowman's capsules has pore
- Filtration based on size of pores
- Blood cells and plasma proteins too large to pass through pores
- Filtrate that enter Bowman's capsule and then PCT has both nutrient and wastes as well as "plenty" of water
Tubular reabsorption
- takes place in PCT
- PCT 1st
- Most of water, nutrients, and electrolytes reabsorbed from filtrate and returned to blood stream to come in contact with filtrate
Loop of Henle
- Thinnest part of nephron
- Counter current mechanism which takes place here further concentrates filtrate
Tubular secretion
- Takes place in DCT
- More wastes are secreted into filtrate in DCT from blood
- Filtrate now enters CT

CT - about a million - join together to form ureter. Filtrate in ureter is referred to as urine

Urinary system:
Ureter: 2 narrow tubes that transport urine formed in kidney to urinary bladder by peristalsis
Urinary system:
Urinary bladder: Hollow muscular organ in pelvic cavity
Wall - layers
- Inner - transitional epithelium
- Middle - smooth muscle (destrussor muscle)
- Outer - connective tissue
Urinary bladder function: store and concentrate urine

Micturition - act of voiding urine

Urinary system:
Urethra
Narrow tube that connects the bladder to the outside
Male
- longer
- transport semen and urine
- UTIs less common
Female
- shorter
- transports urine only
- UTIs more common
Urinary system:
Urine
- Predominantly water
- Has urea, creatinine, and uric acid
- Clear, yellow, / amber colored fluid
- About 1 - 2 litter / day
- PH 6

Reproductive System: Can be divided into the internal reproductive organs and the external genitalia. The gonads are the actual organs that produce the gametes. In the male, testes (singular = testis) produce sperm, and in the female, ovaries make eggs.

Reproductive System:
Male
- Testes
- Accessory sex gland
- External genitalia
Lobules contain: 3 - 6 coiled tubes called seminiferous tubules
Seminiferous tubules: Have 3 types of cells
1. Spermatogonium: parent cell for sperms
2. Sertoli cell: provide support for sperm
3. Interstitial cells of Leydig: produce testosterone
Sperm made in testes go to a C shaped structure called epididymis.

Reproductive System:
Accessory sex glands
1. Seminal vesicle

2. Prostate gland- secrete semen
3. Bulbouretheral gland or Cowper's gland
Bulbouretheral gland or Cowper gland- Contributes mucous secretion that provides lubrication during sexual intercourse
Sperm made in testes go to a C shaped structure called epididymis.

Epididymis - sperms are stored and undergo maturation. From the epididymis sperms are taken into pelvic cavity by the ductus deferens/vas deferens.

Reproductive System:
Female:
- Ovaries
- Uterus
- Fallopian tubes
- Mammary glands
- External genitalia

Reproductive System:
Ovaries:
- In pelvic cavity
- Held in place by ligaments
Oogeneseis: Process by which ova (eggs) are made in ovary

Reproductive System: Ovarian cycle
Events that take place in ovary over a 28 days period
Day 1 - day 13
Follicular phase
- 1 follicle in 1 ovary begin to mature
- Maturing follicle secretes estrogen
Day 14
Ovulation
- Release of egg from ovary
- Mature follicle that release the egg is called graafian follicle
Day 15 - day 28
Luteal phase
- Empty follicle begins to shrink
- Shrinking follicle called corpus luteum: secrete progesterone
Day 28
If egg is fertilized - missed period if egg is not fertilized - next period

Reproductive System:
Menarche - 1st- hollow muscular organ in pelvic cavity period
Menopause - cessation of period
Menstruation - periodic discharge of blood, tissue and mucus through vagina

Reproductive System:
Uterus:
- Hollow muscular organ in pelvic cavity
- Site for growth / development of fetus
Parts:
- Fundus
- Body
- Cervix - part of uterus that extends into vagina
Uterus wall - layers
- Inner - endometrium (epithelial tissue)
- Middle - myometrium (smooth muscle)

- Outer - epimetrium (connective tissue)
Endometrium - inner lining of uterus has 2 layers
1. Inner: stratum basalis (makes new functionalis)
2. Outer: stratum functionalis (shed during each period)

Reproductive System:
Events that take place inside uterus over a 28 day period
Day 1 - day 5
Menstruation; periodic discharge of blood tissue and mucus through vagina
Day 6 - day 14
Proliferative phase: repair of endometrium
Day 15 - day 28
Secretony phase: thickening of endometrium in anti apation of receiving a fertilized egg

Reproductive System:
Fallopian tube: 2 narrow tubes that connect uterus to ovaries Function:
- Site where fertilization takes place (fusion of sperm and eggs)
Parts:
- Isthmus - part of tube that extends into uterus
- Ampulla - widest section of tube
- Infundibulum - distal end
- Fimbriae - fingerlike extensions at distal end
Fertilization:
- Fusion of sperm and egg
- Takes place in fallopian tube
Fertilized egg called zygote goes through repeated mitotic divisions called cleavage
- Cluster of cells called blastula
- Cells rearrange themselves into 3 layers called germ layers

Good Luck on your test!

If any questions or to let us know how we can do better, please feel to contact us at email: hesia2prep@hotmail.com or call:
832-848-0314

ABOUT THE AUTHOR

My name is Tanisha Wilson, I live in the great state of Texas and a pre-Nursing student. I decided to write to this study guide to help fellow students from over and under studying for the HESI A2 Admission Exam. Good luck in your educational pursuits.

CPSIA information can be obtained at www.ICGtesting.com
Printed in the USA
LVOW092055031212

309907LV00026B/2163/P